LMRVT

CLINICIAN MANUAL

LESSAC-MADSEN RESONANT VOICE THERAPY

Katherine Verdolini Abbott, Ph.D., CCC-SLP
Developer and author of "Lessac-Madsen Resonant Voice Therapy"

"This manual may be used as a guide for clinicians who have completed formal training in Lessac-Madsen Resonant Voice Therapy with Dr. Verdolini Abbott or a person she has designated. The material may also be used by patients, educators, and clinicians for informational and educational purposes. However, no individual may use the materials for clinical work, or claim to use the materials for clinical work, without formal training by Dr. Verdolini Abbott or a person she has designated. Such use will constitute an ethical breach and may be pursued under legal auspices."

Dedicated to Professor Arthur Lessac and Dr. Mark Madsen, whose work inspired many parts of the program and to whom I am perpetually indebted.

PLURAL PUBLISHING INC.

Contents

Lessac-Madsen Resonant Voice Therapy (LMRVT)

Note:

This manual is intended for use in voice therapy provided by a licensed speech-language pathologist trained in Lessac Madsen Resonant Voice Therapy (LMRVT) by Dr. Katherine Verdolini Abbott or another individual whom she has appointed. Clinical use of the materials by any other individual is strictly prohibited by the author.

The manual may also be used by educators and students who wish to obtain an overview of the approach and its materials. However, application of the approach or materials to clinical situations without the requisite training is prohibited.

The materials contained herein are not intended to treat or diagnose any condition.

Lessac-Madsen Resonant Voice Therapy (LMRVT) Protocol

Protocol

Schematic representation, prototypical LMRVT Program (30-45 minute sessions; leaving 5 min for initial "check-in" at beginning of each session and 5 min for home instructions at end of each session). See below and next pages for further information. Note that clinician has discretion to change order of items and number of sessions in which items are used. The only requirement is that all items on the Table must be addressed at some point during the program. Also the use and duration of break between back-to-back sessions is at the clinician's discretion.

	Intake Hygiene (30-45 min)	Stretches (5-10 min)	RV Core (5-10 min)	RV Chant (5-10 min)	RV "VC" (5-10 min)	RV "Mini" ("VC" 5-min)	RV "Messa di voce" (5-10 min)	Converse (5-20 min)	OwnTx (15-20 min)
I	✓	(✓)	(✓)						
II		✓	✓	✓	✓			C1	
III		✓	✓	✓	✓	✓		C2	
IV		✓	✓		✓	(✓)	✓	C1+2	
V		✓	✓		✓	(✓)	✓	C3	
VI		✓	✓			(✓)	✓	C4	
VII		✓	✓				✓	C5	
VIII		✓	✓					C6	✓

C1 = normal conversation;
C2 = quiet conversation on telephone, dictaphone, or other as relevant for patient;
C3 = loud voice (over distance) as relevant for patient;
C4 = speech in background noise as relevant to patient;
C5 = emotional speech as relevant to patient;
C6 = "challenge" conversation.

Session 1: History

Demographics : *(May use alternative form)*

Age: ________ Gender: ____________

Occupation: ______________________________________

History *(May use alternative form)*

Symptoms: ______________________________________

____

Circumstances surrounding onset (illness, voice use, stress, etc.): ______________

____

Clinical course since onset (factors aggravating, improving condition): ______________

____

Medical conditions and medications:______________________

Current ENT (including Dx): ______________________

Current general medical/surgical: ______________________

Past ENT: ______________________

Past general medical/surgical: ______________________

Hearing (self and environment): ______________________

Importance of voice problem
(0 = least important thing in the world; 10 = most important thing in the world):______

Motivation for voice therapy
(0 = absolutely not motivated; 10 = extreme motivation):______

Impressions:

(Must complete; copy into patient manual)

Global severity
(per patient; 0 = catastrophic voice;
10 = exquisitely excellent voice; indicate with "X"; indicate clinician rating with check):

10	
9	
8	
7	
6	
5	
4	
3	
2	
1	
0	

Therapy Planning

(Must complete; copy into patient manual)

Likely contributing factors to onset and maintenance of voice problem:

(1) ______________________________

____

(2) ______________________________

____

(3) ______________________________

____

(4) ______________________________

____

(5) ______________________________

____

Goals:

(1) Functional (per patient): ______________________________

____

(2) Medical (per MD): ______________________________

____

(3) Biomechanical (per SLP): ______________________________

____

Treatment program:

Treatment type: ______________________________

How often: ______________________________

How many sessions/weeks: ______________________________

Prognosis:

____

____

❑ Patient history ✐ *(copy into patient manual)*

❑ About LMRVT *(see patient manual)*

❑ Voice care: Summary of recommendations ✐ *(copy from patient manual):*

- ◆ Hydration
  - ❖ Water:
  - ❖ Steam/vapor:
  - ❖ Medication:
- ◆ LPR/Smoking
  - ❖ Behavioral tx:
  - ❖ Drugs:
- ◆ Voice use: screaming, hollering, background noise:

❑ Description of vocal fold vibration, injury, and fatigue using visual aids

Note: *If Session 2 is not initiated same day, proceed to "Basic Training Gesture" exercises (through "m" words and phrases) for Session 2, on the first day of treatment. Include in home program.*

Session 2:

If Session 2 is on different day from Session 1:

- ❑ How was your voice this past week?
- ❑ Patient evaluation of compliance with instructions from Session 1.
  - ◆ None
  - ◆ Somewhat
  - ◆ Quite a bit
  - ◆ Complete
- ❑ Show me exercises (time permitting).
- ❑ Show me special task.

Stretches

- ❑ Completed

RV Core Exercises: BTG

- ❑ "mmmmm" - (with questions; do you feel vibrations in front of face? Is voice easy?)
- ❑ "mmmmm" – x ± 10 (w/ Qs)

Explorations first session only (neg. pract. w/ Qs; /m/)

- ❑ Tighten/loosen lip
- ❑ Tighten/loosen jaw
- ❑ Tighten/loosen throat
- ❑ Tighten/loosen all

Questions:

Do you feel vibrations in the front of your face?

Is voice easy?

Explorations all sessions

- ❑ "mmmmm" – explore making vibrations wider and narrower
- ❑ "mmmmm" – explore making vibrations narrower and narrower, and voice easier and easier
- ❑ "mmmmm" – explore what happens to vibrations shifting tongue in mouth
- ❑ "mmmmm" – explore what happens to vibrations gliding through pitch range; sustain pitch in range where vibrations are strongest, voice easiest (not about "optimal pitch" but rather awareness)
- ❑ "mmmmm" – sustain comfortable pitch and imagine pitch is increasing, but it's not; notice shift in vibrations

- ❑ Definition of RV to patient (any time you have these sensations, you're doing something good for your vocal folds; it's like "medicine;" it can sound different but if you can answer "yes" to these two questions, you're doing it "right"):
  - ◆ Vibrations in the front of your face
  - ◆ Easy

- ❑ **RV Core Exercises: Words**

  Notice if you feel forward vibrations on the "m"s and "n"s (no "trying;" you're the "witness"):

> ***Here and throughout program, training maintains focus on sensory consequences of phonation (anterior vibrations, easy voice), using exploratory is "Scan-gel-show-tell---negative practice."***

Mention	Middle
Moon	Modern
Mundane	Morgan
Man	Marine
Mum	Machine
Motion	Mean
Mon (angahela)	Maiden

- ❑ **RV Core Exercises: Phrases**

The machine is broken.	Morgan likes ice cream.
The moon is out tonight.	I have motion sickness.
Put me in the middle.	

RV Chant

- ❑ /mi mi mi mi mi mi/ (one pitch). Now you do it. Do you feel the vibrations? Is voice easy? Now see if you feel the same vibrations, and the same ease, as we put voiceless sounds in the middle, and as we gradually increase inflection. Repeat after me:
- ❑ /mi mi pi pi mi mi/ (one pitch; to criterion).
- ❑ Meet me Peter, meet me (one pitch; to criterion)
- ❑ Meet me Peter, meet me. (gradually increase inflection over several trials, to criterion).
- ❑ Hi, my name's Peter. What am I supposed to do this afternoon? (Response, with natural inflection: Meet me, Peter, meet me!).

- ❑ /ma ma ma ma ma ma/ (one pitch; to criterion).
- ❑ /ma ma pa pa ma ma/ (one pitch; to criterion).
- ❑ Mama, papa, mama (one pitch; to criterion).
- ❑ Mama, papa, mama (gradually increase inflection over several trials, to criterion).
- ❑ So, what does the child say looking from her mother to her father to her mother again? (Response, with natural inflection: Mama, Papa, Mama!).
- ❑ /mu mu mu mu mu mu/ (one pitch; to criterion).
- ❑ /mu mu pu pu mu mu/ (one pitch; to criterion).
- ❑ Mooching pooches, mooching (one pitch; to criterion).
- ❑ Mooching pooches, mooching (gradually increase inflection over several trials, to criterion).
- ❑ So, what do you think you are going to be doing this afternoon? (Response, with natural inflection: Mooching pooches, mooching!).

RV Vocal Communicator

- ❑ Conversational speech: regular conversation, in quiet, at short distance, in the treatment room. Encourage "real" communication-—using "m-hmmm" etc. responses.

Discharge

Real life management (examples):

- ❑ RV fairly quietly at first; later will teach loud RV but don't use until then.
- ❑ Explain your voice work to appropriate family, friends, peers, and/or colleagues and ask for their support.
- ❑ Get people's attention by moving closer to them; if teacher, turn lights on/off, raise hand till you get attention, etc.
- ❑ Other:

Daily voice work program

- ❑ Each time you come in from now on, I will ask you to show me your exercises so we can troubleshoot them.
- ❑ I will fill out a template for your daily voice work. Then you fill out one sheet for every day of practice. Bring the whole booklet back for review each session. (Optional, recommended: Provide patient with CD of exercises.)[1]
- ❑ When you come back next week, be able to do do ______________with your voice!

---

[1] *Clinician works with patient to determine what exercises, and when. Usually, home program will reflect exercises done during proceeding session. Exercises should be part of life, not separate from it, and should not require "time out."*

Session 3

- ❑ How was your voice this past week?
- ❑ Patient evaluation of compliance based on homework
  - ◆ None
  - ◆ Somewhat
  - ◆ Quite a bit
  - ◆ Complete
- ❑ Show me exercises (time permitting)
- ❑ Show me special task

Stretches

RV Core Exercises: BTG

- ❑ "nnnnnn"
- ❑ "nnnnnn" - x + 10 (w/ Qs)
- ❑ "nnnnnnn";"gegegege" - explore making vibrations wider and narrower.
- ❑ "rrrrrr";"llllll" - explore making vibrations narrower and narrower, and voice easier and easier.
- ❑ "zzzzz";"vvvvv" - explore what happens to vibrations shifting tongue in mouth.
- ❑ "ngngngng";"mmmmm" - explore what happens to vibrations gliding through pitch range; sustain pitch in range where vibrations are strongest, voice easiest (not about "optimal pitch" but rather awareness).

❑ RV Core Exercises: Words

Room	Laugh	Neck	Boring
Visit	Raining	Zero	Lemon
Naughty	Vague	Mug	Roam
Zorro	Mom		

❑ **RV Core Exercises: Phrases**

(note: scales on "mmmmm" + vowels may be substituted for phrases)

Will you visit me today?

It's raining outside.

I love lemon flavoring.

The boy was naughty.

Don't be so vague.

RV chant

❑ /no no no no no no/ (one pitch; to criterion).

❑ /no no to to no no/ (one pitch; to criterion).

❑ No no, Toto, no no! (one pitch; to criterion).

❑ No no, Toto, no no! (gradually increase inflection over several trials, to criterion).

❑ Would you like a pie in the face? (Response, with natural inflection: No no, Toto, no no!).

❑ /zi zi zi zi zi zi/ (one pitch; to criterion).

❑ /zi zi si si zi zi/ (one pitch; to criterion).

❑ Ziti Sissy, ziti! (one pitch; to criterion).

❑ Ziti Sissy, ziti! (gradually increase inflection over several trials, to criterion).

❑ I'm your waitress. What would you like to order? (Response, with natural inflection: Ziti, Sissy, ziti!).

❑ /vu vu vu vu vu vu/ (one pitch; to criterion).

❑ /vu vu fu fu vu vu/ (one pitch; to criterion).

❑ Voodoo, foolish voodoo! (one pitch; to criterion).

❑ Voodoo, foolish voodoo! (gradually increase inflection over several trials, to criterion).

❑ What religion does your friend practice? (Response, with natural inflection: Voodoo, foolish voodoo).

- ❑ **RV Vocal Communicator**
  - ◆ "m-hmmm," "really," "right," "yeah," "no"

RV Mini

- ❑ Identify strategies to pull out of old voice to resonant voice: Excusing oneself from the room altogether/switch gears at a phrase boundary or in the middle of a phrase/change positions slightly, take a breath, and continue on with the next phrase in RV, etc.
- ❑ Patient counts 1-5 in old voice. Then, patient pulls out and counts 6-10 in RV.
- ❑ Conversation with mini (switching between old and new voice as indicated by thumbs up and thumbs down).

RV Conversation

- ❑ Quiet conversation, speaking into a device at close range (e.g., telephone, dictaphone, or other as relevant for the patient).

Discharge (If Session 4 is not on same day as Session 3)

- ❑ Home program
- ❑ When you come back next week, be able to do ______ with your voice!

Session 4

(If Session 4 is not on same day as Session 3:)

- ❑ How was your voice this past week?
- ❑ Patient evaluation of compliance based on homework
  - ◆ None
  - ◆ Somewhat
  - ◆ Quite a bit
  - ◆ Complete
- ❑ Show me exercises (time permitting).
- ❑ Show me special task.

RV Core Exercises: BTG

- ❑ "mmmmm"
- ❑ "mmmmm" – x + 10 (w/ Qs)
- ❑ "mmmmm";"gegegege" – explore making vibrations wider and narrower.
- ❑ "zzzzzzz";"ngngngngng" – explore making vibrations narrower and narrower, and voice easier and easier.
- ❑ "rrrrrrr";"vvvvv" – explore what happens to vibrations shifting tongue in mouth.
- ❑ "nnnnnnn";"lllllll" – explore what happens to vibrations gliding through pitch range; sustain pitch in range where vibrations are strongest, voice easiest (not about "optimal pitch" but rather awareness).

❑ RV Core Exercises: Words

Lodge	Zip	Murmur	Notice	Rug
Mood	Raw	Venture	Little	Rate
Van	Xerox	Nepal	Meringue	

❑ RV Core Exercises: Phrases (note: scales on nasals + vowels may be substituted for phrases)

The little girl is lost.

My rug is white.

Nepal is a beautiful country.

Don't venture beyond the house.

Please make a Xerox copy.

RV Messa di Voce

- ❑ Practice on "/mmmjjjiiiii/", "/mmmjjjaaaaa/" and "/mmmjjjuuuuu/" (crescendo over a count of 4; descrescendo over a count of 4).

- ❑ Practice the list:

Hey	Hey	Hey	Hey	Hey	Hey	Hey
Yo	Yo	Yo	Yo	Yo	Yo	Yo
Hey Joe	Hey Joe	Hey Joe	Hey Joe	Hey Joe	Hey Joe	Hey Joe

- ❑ Practice the list:

Venture	Venture	Venture	Venture	Venture	Venture	Venture
Zip	Zip	Zip	Zip	Zip	Zip	Zip
Nepal	Nepal	Nepal	Nepal	Nepal	Nepal	Nepal
Meringue	Meringue	Meringue	Meringue	Meringue	Meringue	Meringue
Little	Little	Little	Little	Little	Little	Little
Notice	Notice	Notice	Notice	Notice	Notice	Notice
Rung	Rung	Rung	Rung	Rung	Rung	Rung
Van	Van	Van	Van	Van	Van	Van
Xerox	Xerox	Xerox	Xerox	Xerox	Xerox	Xerox
Murmur	Murmur	Murmur	Murmur	Murmur	Murmur	Murmur
Mood	Mood	Mood	Mood	Mood	Mood	Mood
Raw	Raw	Raw	Raw	Raw	Raw	Raw
Lodge	Lodge	Lodge	Lodge	Lodge	Lodge	Lodge
Rate	Rate	Rate	Rate	Rate	Rate	Rate

RV Vocal Communicator Combined with Mini

- "yeah," "really," "right," "no", "m-hmmmm."

RV Conversation

- ❑ Regular conversation, in quiet, at short distance, in the tx room + quiet conversation, speaking into a device at close range (e.g., telephone, dictaphone, or other as relevant for the patient).

Discharge

- ❑ Home program
- ❑ When you come back next week, be able to do ____________ with your voice!

Session 5

- ❑ How was your voice this past week?
- ❑ Patient evaluation of compliance based on homework
    - ◆ None
    - ◆ Somewhat
    - ◆ Quite a bit
    - ◆ Complete
- ❑ Show me exercises (time permitting).
- ❑ Show me special task.

Stretches

RV Core Exercises: BTG

- ❑ "vvvvvvv"
- ❑ "vvvvvvv" - x + 10 (w/ Qs)
- ❑ "vvvvvvv";"nnnnnnn" - explore making vibrations wider and narrower "gegegege"; "ngngngngng" - explore making vibrations narrower and narrower, and voice easier and easier.
- ❑ "zzzzzz";"rrrrrrr" - explore what happens to vibrations shifting tongue in mouth.
- ❑ "mmmmm";"lllllll" - explore what happens to vibrations gliding through pitch range; sustain pitch in range where vibrations are strongest, voice easiest (not about "optimal pitch" but rather awareness).

❑ RV Core Exercises: Words

Lawn	Met	Verbal	Vote
Remain	Middle	Love	Nanny
Swimming	Zombie	Dancing	Zoo
Rain	Near		

❏ **RV Core Exercises: Phrases** (note: scales on nasals + vowels may be substituted for phrases)

The zoo is closed today.

My brother is so verbal.

Let's go swimming.

I have to vote later.

You are dancing with him?

RV Messa di Voce

❏ Practice on "/nnnjjjiiiii/", "nnngggjjjaaaaa/", "/vvvjjjuuuuu/" (crescendo over a count of 4; decrescendo over a count of 4).

❏ Practice the list:

Hey	Hey	Hey	Hey	Hey	Hey	Hey
Yo	Yo	Yo	Yo	Yo	Yo	Yo
Hey Joe	Hey Joe	Hey Joe	Hey Joe	Hey Joe	Hey Joe	Hey Joe

❏ Practice the list:

Dancing	Dancing	Dancing	Dancing	Dancing	Dancing	Dancing
Rain	Rain	Rain	Rain	Rain	Rain	Rain
Remain	Remain	Remain	Remain	Remain	Remain	Remain
Zoo	Zoo	Zoo	Zoo	Zoo	Zoo	Zoo
Verbal	Verbal	Verbal	Verbal	Verbal	Verbal	Verbal
Love	Love	Love	Love	Love	Love	Love
Swimming	Swimming	Swimming	Swimming	Swimming	Swimming	swimming
Vote	Vote	Vote	Vote	Vote	Vote	Vote
Met	Met	Met	Met	Met	Met	Met
Nanny	Nanny	Nanny	Nanny	Nanny	Nanny	Nanny
Lawn	Lawn	Lawn	Lawn	Lawn	Lawn	Lawn
Middle	Middle	Middle	Middle	Middle	Middle	Middle
Near	Near	Near	Near	Near	Near	Near
Zombie	Zombie	Zombie	Zombie	Zombie	Zombie	Zombie

RV Vocal Communicator Combined with Mini:

- "yeah," "really," "right," "no", "m-hmmmm"

❏ Conversation: Speaking loudly over a distance (e.g. classroom scenario).

❏ (If Session 6 is not on same day as Session 5: When you come back next week, be able to do ____________ with your voice!

RV Conversation

❏ Speaking loudly over a distance (e.g. classroom , courtroom, church, sports field, or other scenario appropriate to the patient.

Discharge (If Session 6 is not on same day as Session 5)

❏ Home program

❏ When you come back next week, be able to do ______ with your voice!

Session 6

(If Session 6 is not on same day as Session 5:)

- ❑ How was your voice this past week?
- ❑ Patient evaluation of compliance based on homework
  - ◆ None
  - ◆ Somewhat
  - ◆ Quite a bit
  - ◆ Complete
- ❑ Show me exercises (time permitting).
- ❑ Show me special task.

Stretches

RV Core Exercises: BTG

- ❑ "zzzzzz"
- ❑ "zzzzzz" - x + 10 (w/ Qs)
- ❑ "zzzzzz";"rrrrrrr" - explore making vibrations wider and narrower "gegegege";"ngngngngng" - explore making vibrations narrower and narrower, and voice easier and easier.
- ❑ "nnnnnnnn";"vvvvvvvvvvv" - explore what happens to vibrations shifting tongue in mouth.
- ❑ "llllllllll";"mmmmm" - explore what happens to vibrations gliding through pitch range; sustain pitch in range where vibrations are strongest, voice easiest (not about "optimal pitch" but rather awareness).

❑ RV Core Exercises: Words

Zap	Rest	Lamp
Singing	Nerd	Tong
Mate	Volume	Meet
Knock	Zone	Romp
Loop	Victim	

❑ RV Core Exercises: Phrases (note: scales on nasals + vowels may be substituted for phrases)

We left the lamp in the window.	Let's meet at 2:30
Turn the volume down.	Take a rest before we continue.
The bird is singing.	

RV Messa di Voce

- ❏ "/zzzjjjiiiii/";"/zzzjjjaaaaa)";"/zzzjjjuuuuu/" (crescendo over a count of 4: decrescendo over a count of 4).
- ❏ Practice the list:

Hey	Hey	Hey	Hey	Hey	Hey	Hey
Yo	Yo	Yo	Yo	Yo	Yo	Yo
Hey Joe	Hey Joe	Hey Joe	Hey Joe	Hey Joe	Hey Joe	Hey Joe

- ❏ Practice the list:

Zap	Zap	Zap	Zap	Zap	Zap	Zap
Mate	Mate	Mate	Mate	Mate	Mate	Mate
Singing	Singing	Singing	Singing	Singing	Singing	Singing
Knock	Knock	Knock	Knock	Knock	Knock	Knock
Romp	Romp	Romp	Romp	Romp	Romp	Romp
Zone	Zone	Zone	Zone	Zone	Zone	Zone
Meet	Meet	Meet	Meet	Meet	Meet	Meet
Volume	Volume	Volume	Volume	Volume	Volume	Volume
Tong	Tong	Tong	Tong	Tong	Tong	Tong
Lamp	Lamp	Lamp	Lamp	Lamp	Lamp	Lamp
Rest	Rest	Rest	Rest	Rest	Rest	Rest
Victim	Victim	Victim	Victim	Victim	Victim	Victim
Loop	Loop	Loop	Loop	Loop	Loop	Loop
Nerd	Nerd	Nerd	Nerd	Nerd	Nerd	Nerd

RV Mini

- ❏ Completed

RV Conversation

- ❏ Speaking in background noise: Simulate relevant situation and record so patient can hear effect of noise later.

Discharge

- ❏ Home program
- ❏ When you come back next week, be able to do ____________ with your voice!

Session 7

- ❑ How was your voice this past week?
- ❑ Patient evaluation of compliance based on homework
  - ◆ None
  - ◆ Somewhat
  - ◆ Quite a bit
  - ◆ Complete
- ❑ Show me exercises (time permitting).
- ❑ Show me special task.

Stretches

RV Core Exercises: BTG

- ❑ "rrrrrrr"
- ❑ "rrrrrrr" - x + 10 (w/ Qs)
- ❑ "rrrrrrr";"lllllllll" - explore making vibrations wider and narrower "vvvvvvv";"nnnnnn" - explore making vibrations narrower and narrower, and voice easier and easier.
- ❑ "gegegege";"mmmmm" - explore what happens to vibrations shifting tongue in mouth.
- ❑ "ngngngng";"zzzzzzzz" - explore what happens to vibrations gliding through pitch range; sustain pitch in range where vibrations are strongest, voice easiest (not about "optimal pitch" but rather awareness).

❑ **RV Core Exercises: Words**

Lit	Metal	Nerve	Voodoo	Zebra
Nonsense	Log	Rugged	Zodiac	Working
Monday	Playing	Race	Vigor	

❑ **RV Core Exercises: Phrases** (note: scales on nasals + vowels may be substituted for phrases)

You are always working.

That's nonsense.

Monday is the first day of the work week.

The race starts tomorrow.

What is your zodiac sign?

RV Messa di voce

- ❑ Practice on "/wwwjjjiiiii/";"/ jjjaaaaa/";"gegege/jjjuuuuu/" crescendo over a count of 4; decrescendo over a count of 4)
- ❑ Practice the list:

Hey	Hey	Hey	Hey	Hey	Hey	Hey
Yo	Yo	Yo	Yo	Yo	Yo	Yo
Hey Joe	Hey Joe	Hey Joe	Hey Joe	Hey Joe	Hey Joe	Hey Joe

- ❑ Practice the list:

Zebra	Zebra	Zebra	Zebra	Zebra	Zebra	Zebra
Voodoo	Voodoo	Voodoo	Voodoo	Voodoo	Voodoo	Voodoo
Working	Working	Working	Working	Working	Working	working
Monday	Monday	Monday	Monday	Monday	Monday	Monday
Lit	Lit	Lit	Lit	Lit	Lit	Lit
Playing	Playing	Playing	Playing	Playing	Playing	Playing
Vigor	Vigor	Vigor	Vigor	Vigor	Vigor	Vigor
Rugged	Rugged	Rugged	Rugged	Rugged	Rugged	Rugged
Nerve	Nerve	Nerve	Nerve	Nerve	Nerve	Nerve
Zodiac	Zodiac	Zodiac	Zodiac	Zodiac	Zodiac	Zodiac
Nonsense	Nonsense	Nonsense	Nonsense	Nonsense	Nonsense	Nonsense
Metal	Metal	Metal	Metal	Metal	Metal	Metal
Log	Log	Log	Log	Log	Log	Log
Race	Race	Race	Race	Race	Race	Race

RV Conversation

- ❑ Emotional topic as relevant for the patient.

Discharge (If Session 8 is not on same day as Session 7)

- ❑ Home program
- ❑ When you come back next week, be able to do ______ with your voice!

Session 8

(If Session 8 is not on same day as Session 7:)

❑ How was your voice this past week?

❑ Patient evaluation of compliance based on homework

- None
- Somewhat
- Quite a bit
- Complete

❑ Show me exercises (time permitting).

❑ Show me special task.

Stretches

RV Core Exercises: BTG

❑ "zzzzzz"

❑ "zzzzzz" – x + 10 (w/ Qs)

❑ "zzzzzz";"mmmmm" – explore making vibrations wider and narrower.

❑ "llllllllll";"ngngngngng" – explore making vibrations narrower and narrower, and voice easier and easier.

❑ "rrrrrrr";"nnnnnnnnn" – explore what happens to vibrations shifting tongue in mouth.

❑ "vvvvvvv";"gegegege" – explore what happens to vibrations gliding through pitch range; sustain pitch in range where vibrations are strongest, voice easiest (not about "optimal pitch" but rather awareness).

❑ **RV Core Exercises: Words**

Zeus	Load	Return	Talking	Knaw
Nod	zest	Rim	Much	Main
Verizon	Vat	Sitting	Lean	

❑ **RV Core Exercises: Phrases** (note: scales on nasals + vowels may be substituted for phrases)

Stop talking during the movie.

Zeus is a Greek God.

Don't take too much salt.

Please return home soon.

Where's the main floor?

RV Conversation

- ❏ "Challenge" trials

Final Discharge

- ❏ Evaluate functional goals with patient.
- ❏ Discharge planning
    - ◆ Practice from here on out (e.g. exercises from Session 8 once daily x 1 wk; three times weekly x 1 wk; once weekly from there on out; if ground is lost, increase practice till back to optimum).
    - ◆ What to do if you get hoarse (due to URI or voice use)? (BTG, words, and phrases quietly, with extreme RV, for several minutes throughout the day; go easy on voice; hydrate; if not returned to baseline in 72 hr or less, seek evaluation by ENT immediately).